SURAT SHABD YOGA
The Yoga of the Celestial Sound

An Introduction for Western Readers

SURAT SHABD YOGA
The Yoga of the Celestial Sound

An Introduction for Western Readers

BY KIRPAL SINGH

The Unity of Man Series

Berkeley
Images Press

Books by Kirpal Singh

The Jap Ji: The Message of Guru Nanak
Prayer
Spirituality
Naam or Word
Baba Jaimal Singh: His Life and Teachings
The Wheel of Life: The Law of Action and Reaction
The Crown of Life
Godman
Spiritual Elixir
The Mystery of Death
Morning Talks
The Night Is A Jungle
Heart-To-Heart Talks

© 1975, Images Press
P.O. Box 9444, Berkeley, California
LCCN 75-42816; ISBN 9600374-4-6

This book was abridged and edited from the *Crown of Life* by Robert Leverant, Unity of Man Series Editor; all or portions may be reproduced by writing the publisher for acknowledgement.

Dedicated
to the Almighty God
working through all Masters who have come
and Baba Sawan Singh Ji Maharaj
at whose lotus feet
the writer imbibed sweet elixir of
Holy Naam—the Word

PREFACE

IN THIS AGE OF PUBLISHING, THERE IS NO DEARTH OF BOOKS ON YOGA. However, if one scrutinizes them carefully, one finds that the majority fall short in one direction or another. They either treat it as primarily a system of *asanas* and physical exercises, or as an abstract and highly monistic system of thought, positing the unity of all existence and the ultimate oneness of the individual soul and the Oversoul. In either case, the view of yoga that we gather is an incomplete one, reducing it from a practical mode of spiritual transcendence and union with the Absolute, to a system of physical culture or school (or group of schools) of philosophy.

To avoid the possibility of such error, the ultimate aim of all yoga, at-one-ment with the Supreme Lord, has been kept as a focusing point for all discussions in this study. All the important forms, ancient and modern, are briefly taken up in turn, their practices explained and discussed, and the extent to which each can lead us toward the final goal evaluated. This last is perhaps the most easily misunderstood and the most widely confused aspect of a comparative study of yoga. It is a characteristic of mystic experience that the soul as it ascends to a plane higher than the one to which it is accustomed, tends (in the absence of superior guidance) to mistake the higher plane as the very highest, the Absolute Realm. And so we find that most yogas, while taking us up to certain point on the inner journey, mistake this for its end, and for a relative validity claim for themselves an absolute one.

The only way by which we can effectively evaluate the comparative spiritual value of each yogic form is by adopting as a standard the very highest form of yoga. This standard is provided by the *Surat Shabd Yoga* also known as *Sant Mat* (or the path of the *Sants* or Masters). By following its practices under proper guidance, its adepts have reached realms not known to other mystic schools, and have finally merged with the Supreme Lord in His Absolute, Nameless and Formless State. They have, in their compositions, repeatedly affirmed the incomparable superiority of this *Yoga of the Sound Current,* while describing through direct inner perception the varying spiritual range of other yogas.

Once a seeker can begin to grasp the perspectives on comparative mysticism which Surat Shabd Yoga can provide, he will, I believe, find this extremely complex subject becoming progressively clearer to him. He will see that the contradictions which disturb so many when they first undertake a comparative study of mysticism are not essential to mystic experience as such, but are the result of a confusion of a relative truth with an absolute one. He will no longer be tempted to evade the issue of spirituality by dismissing it as a mere remnant of old superstition and black magic, but will begin to see it as a kind of timeless inner science with its own unchanging laws and varying modes of operations. And above all, he will, I hope, realize that mergence with the Supreme Lord is no mere day-dream or hypothetical postulate of a monistic school of philosophy, but a living possibility whose realization is the true end of human existence and whose attainment, given the right guidance, the right method and the right effort, lies within the reach of all, irrespective of age, sex, race or creed.

Kirpal Singh

CONTENTS

Preface 7

Part 1 THE YOGAS
    I. The Philosophical Background 13
    II. Yoga: Its Aims and Assumptions 14
    III. Samadhi 16
    IV. The Origins of Yoga 18
    V. The Derivative Yogas 20
    VI. The Drawbacks to Karma and Jnana Yoga .. 23
    VII. The Limitation of Bhakti Yoga 25

Part 2 SURAT SHABD YOGA
    I. Scriptural References 31
    II. The Shabd Or Word 34
    III. The Easy Way: Comparisons & Difficulties . 35
    IV. The Living Master 38
    V. Recognizing A Living Master 41
    VI. Sadachar: Charity 44
    VII. Sadachar: Chastity 46
    VIII. Sadhna: Spiritual Discipline 49

IX. The Radiant Form of the Master 51
X. Love and the Lover's Relationship 54
XI. A Perfect Science 57

Appendix

1. Chart of the Chakras or Plexuses 61
2. Some Yamas and Niyamas 62
3. A Daily Spiritual Diary 63
4. Traditional Hatha Yoga Foods 64
5. Chart of the Planes of Creation 65

Afterword: Yoga and the Outer Sciences 69

PART 1
THE YOGAS

I. THE PHILOSOPHICAL BACKGROUND

IT HAS BEEN TAUGHT SINCE TIME IMMEMORIAL BY THE INDIAN SAGES THAT BEHIND THE APPARENT SELF OF WHICH WE ARE CONSCIOUS IN EVERYDAY EXISTENCE, THE SELF THAT SHIRKS PAIN AND SEEKS PLEASURE, THAT CHANGES FROM MOMENT TO MOMENT AND IS SUBJECT TO THE EFFECT OF TIME AND SPACE, THERE IS THE PERMANENT "SELF," THE *ATMAN*. This Atman forms the basic reality, the final substance, the essence of essences, and it is in the light of its being that all else assumes meaning. Similarly, the Indian mystics have analyzed the nature of the Universe. Seen from the surface, they say, our world appears to be a queer composition of contradictory elements. Faced with these contradictions, man is compelled to look for a Creator who holds the opposing forces in balance and represents permanence behind the flux of existence. As he penetrates deeper and deeper, he discovers that the contradictions are only apparent, not real: that far from being opposed in nature, they are differentiated manifestations of the same Power, and that they are not even "manifestations" properly, but are illusions of the mind which are dispelled in the light of realization.

These two insights are basic to Indian thought, and on closer examination will be seen to be not separate, but one. If behind the changing, time-ridden self, there be an eternal, changeless and timeless One, and if behind the flux of mutability of the creation as we normally know it, there be an

Absolute Immutable Reality, then the two must be related and must in fact be the same. How can there be two Absolutes?

The moment we realize this truth about the nature of Self and Overself, or the One Truth about the nature of Reality, the problem that inevitably poses itself is: why do we in everyday existence experience the world in terms of duality and plurality, feeling ourselves separate from each other and from life in general, and what may be the means for transcending this constriction of ourselves and merging into the Ocean of Consciousness that is our essential state?

The answer to the first part of this question is that the spirit, in its downward descent, gets enveloped in fold upon fold of mental and material apparatus which compel it to experience life in terms of their limitations, until, no longer conscious of its own inherent nature, the soul identifies itself with their realm of time and space—*nam-rup-prapanch*. The answer to the second part is that the soul can bear witness to itself, provided it can divest itself of its limiting adjuncts. The many forms of yoga "are various methods which have been developed by the Indian sages for accomplishing this process of disentanglement or spiritual involution." Yoga, in brief, stands for a technique of reorientation and reintegration of the spirit in man, the lost continent of his true self.

II. YOGA: ITS AIMS AND ASSUMPTIONS

YOGA PRESUPPOSES TWO FACTORS THAT ACCOUNT FOR THE CREATION OF THE WORLD: (1) *ISHWAR* OR GOD AND (2) *AVIDYA* OR MAYA. WHILE THE FORMER IS ALL INTELLIGENT, THE LATTER IS ALTOGETHER UNINTELLIGENT. Man, too, is a combination of these two basic principles. *Jiva* or the individual soul though intrinsically of the same essence as that of God, is encased in mind and matter. The soul, conditioned as it is in the time-space-cause world, has but an imperfect perception and cannot see the reality, the *atman* or the Divine Ground, in which it rests and from which it gets its luminosity.

To free the individual soul from the shackles of mind and matter, yoga insists on (1) concentration, (2) active effort or striving, which involves the performance of devotional exercises and mental discipline. The highest form of matter is *chit*, the unfathomable lake of subliminal impressions, and yoga aims at freeing the inner man or spirit from these fetters. It is the finest and rarefied principle in matter that constitutes chit or the little self (ego) in man. Though in itself it is essentially unconscious, it has also the capacity to contract and expand according to the nature of the body in which it is lodged from time to time, or according to the surrounding circumstances.

This *chit* or mind, though apparently bounded in each individual, is in fact a part of the all-pervading universal mind. The yoga systems aim at transforming the limited and conditioned mind into limitless and unconditioned Universal mind, by developing the *satva* (pure) and by subduing the *rajas* (active) and *tamas* (dense) *gunas* or qualities which compose and determine an individual's personality. In this state, yogins acquire omniscience.

Subliminal impressions in the chit cause desires and interest, which in turn produce potencies, and these lead to personality, thus setting the wheel of the world in perpetual motion. When once the soul is freed from the *chit*, desires, potencies, and personality, it comes into its own, and becomes passionless and depersonalized. This is the great deliverance which yoga promises to yogins. At this severance from the four-fold fetters of the mind, the embodied soul (*jiva*) becomes a freed soul (*atman*), unindividualized, self-luminous, and attains realization as such. "Self-realization" then is the highest aim of yoga.

III. SAMADHI

THE TERM *SAMADHI* IS DERIVED FROM TWO SANSKRIT ROOTS: *SAM* WITH ITS ENGLISH EQUIVALENT "SYN" MEANS "TOGETHER WITH," AND *ADHI* (THE PRIMAL BEING) WITH ITS HEBREW EQUIVALENT OF *ADON* OR *ADONAI* WHICH DENOTES "LORD." The two together, *sam* plus *adhi*, denote a state in which the mind is completely absorbed in the Lord or God. It is a state in which all limiting forms drop away and the individual, with his individuality all dissolved, experiences the great truth *Ayam Athma Brahma*—"I am Thou."

It is the last and culminating stage in the long-drawn-out process of experimental yoga, and may therefore be said to be the efflorescence of the yogic system. Meditation itself gradually develops into samadhi when the contemplator or the meditator loses all thought of himself, and the mind becomes *dhya-rupa*, the very form of his thought. In this state the aspirant is not conscious of any external object save of Consciousness itself, a state of all Bliss or perfect happiness.

This state of identification with the Absolute may be accompanied with consciousness of one's individuality, in which case it is known as *savikalpa samadhi*, or it may not be accompanied with any such consciousness and is then known as *nirvikalpa samadhi*. The former was compared by Sri Ramakrishna to a cotton doll which when put in water gets saturated with it, and the latter to a doll of salt which when immersed in water dissolves and loses itself in it. Of these, nirvikalpa is the higher, for savikalpa, though it greatly widens one's vision, is yet only a preliminary step toward the unconditioned state. Not all yogins can achieve nirvikalpa, and those who do attain it generally do so only once in their life. They thereby finally escape the realm of name and form and become liberated souls. On returning from nirvikalpa, or the unconditioned state, to everyday human consciousness, they live and move as other human beings. But while engaged in worldly duties, they are forever centered in the Divine and are never separate from It. This state of normal activity on the plane of the senses but imbued with God-realization, is designated as *Sehaj Samadhi* or the state of Easy Union.

> *Whether sitting, standing or walking about,*
> *They ever remain in a state of eternal equipoise.*
>
> KABIR

We may also mention yet another form of samadhi, called *Bhava Samadhi,* in which the devotee, lost in devotional music and singing, loses all thought of himself and the world around. This form of samadhi is easy to attain for those of an emotional temperament and affords momentary ecstasy and inner mental relief, but it does not give at-one-ment with the Divine or expand one's consciousness. As such, the term *samadhi* is only loosely applied to it, for it displays none of the central attributes of the super-conscious state, nor is it therefore of much help on the inner spiritual journey.

The state of samadhi is not a stone-like, inert state, or a state of withdrawal similar to that of a tortoise withdrawing into its shell. Each one of us is endowed with a rich inner life, full of untold spiritual gems of which ordinarily we are not conscious in the work-a-day present life of the senses that we usually lead. We can turn inward and expand our vision so as to embrace within its fold not only a cosmic life but even a super-cosmic life as well, extending into vistas beyond the human ken. It is a state of being, a direct perception, an integral experience of the soul. The spiritual experience, though it stands by itself and is beyond the farthest limits of reason, does not however contradict reason, but makes reason perfect.

The one recurring theme in the teachings of all great rishis and mystics has been that their insights are based not on inherited learning, philosophical speculation or logical reasoning, but on first-hand inner experience or *anubhava*—a word whose lucidity of expressiveness defies translation. Yoga, means steadiness of mind, born of *chit-vriti-nirodha* (nullification of mind or elimination from the mind of all mental vibrations), and the term *samadhi,* comprising the two Sanskrit roots *sam* and *adhi,* denotes acceptance, absorption, steadiness in contemplation, or deep inward concentration.

IV. THE ORIGINS OF YOGA

FROM THE *YAJNAVALKYA SMRITI*, WE LEARN THAT HIRANYAGARBHA (BRAHMA) WAS THE ORIGINAL TEACHER OF YOGA. BUT THE YOGA SYSTEM, AS A SYSTEM, WAS FIRST EXPOUNDED BY PATANJALI, THE GREAT THINKER AND PHILOSOPHER, IN HIS *YOGA SUTRAS,* SOMETIME BEFORE THE CHRISTIAN ERA. The yogic system is one of the six schools of Indian philosophy (*Khat Shastras*) that were systematized and developed to set in order Indian thought concerning the cosmos, the individual soul, and their interrelation.

The term *yoga* is derived from the Sanskrit root *yuj* which means meeting, union, communion, consummation, abstraction, realization, absorption or metaphysical philosophizing of the highest type, that promises to bring close proximity between the soul and the Oversoul. PATANJALI defines yoga as elimination of the *vritis* or modulations that always keep surging in the mind-stuff or *chit* in the form of ripples. He calls it *chit vriti nirodha* or the suppression of the vritis, i.e., clearing the mind of the mental oscillations.

> *Chit-vriti nirodha (clearing the mind of the mental oscillations) is the essence of yoga.*
>
> PATANJALI

The *Ashtang Yoga* system of Patanjali is a rigorous discipline involving intense and solitary meditation coupled with physical exercises and postures to discipline and control the mind and the *pranas* or breath currents so as to make them run in a particular manner that may help in subduing the senses. As such, it is meant for the purification of the body and mind, and prepares the way for the beatific vision. It is far from easy to practice. Gaudapada, his progenitor, admitted that to pursue it was like attempting to empty the sea drop by drop with the aid of a blade of grass. If one was to achieve anything substantial in this practice, one had to begin from infancy itself. The first twenty-five years of *brahmcharya* or celibacy were to be utilized in the proper development of one's body and mind, in building up physical and spiritual health capable of withstanding life's rigors. The next twenty-five years, *grehastya*, were to be lived as a householder, as the head of a family, a prop to the old, a supporter to the wife, and a sound teacher to the children. Obligations to society performed, death drawing nearer, and life tasted to the full, one was free to seek its inner meaning and ripe for its understanding. And so, the succeeding twenty-five years were to be spent in *vanprasth*, in the solitude of mountain and forest, until through various sadhnas and strenuous meditation one had gained enlightenment. Now at last one was fit to be called a *sanyasin* and able to devote the last quarter of the century-span as envisaged in the perfect life, to the task of assisting one's fellow men in their search for spiritual freedom.

Even in olden days, the ideal of the four *ashramas* was not an easy one. Little wonder then that yoga was restricted to the chosen few and was not propagated as a course to be followed by the common people, continuing only as a mystery school whose torch was passed on from *guru* (teacher) to *chela* (disciple) in a restricted line. If anything, modern conditions have rendered its pursuit in this form even more difficult and well-nigh impossible. As life has become more complex and the various professions more specialized, men no longer find it possible to devote the first twenty-five years of their life solely to the cultivation of body and mind in preparation for the final quest. They must spend them in schools, colleges and institutes, which employ most of their resources in training them for a career. Nor, with the ever-growing population, is it feasible to expect one-fourth of the members of society—*grehastis*—to provide the means of physical sustenance for the remaining three-quarters, as was once perhaps possible.

As if this were not enough, the integrated eightfold yoga of Patanjali seems to have grown more specialized and complicated with the passage of time. Each of its branches has developed to a point where it almost seems a complete subject in itself. Little wonder then that man, practicing in their various details the various *yamas* (abstentions) and *niyamas* (observances), or mastering the different *asanas* (postures) or learning to control the *pranic* (breath) or *mansic* (mental) energies, begins to imagine that his particular field of specialization is not, as Patanjali envisaged, just a rung in the ladder of the integrated yoga, but yoga itself.

V. THE DERIVATIVE YOGAS

LATER RISHIS AND TEACHERS DERIVED MUCH GUIDANCE FROM PATANJALI, BUT THEIR TEACHINGS IMPLICITLY EMBODY THE RECOGNITION THAT HIS SYSTEM IS TOO EXACTING AND TENDS TO DENY SPIRITUAL ATTAINMENT TO THE AVERAGE MAN. If spirituality must entail a slow ascension through all the rungs of this intricate and involved ladder of yoga, then it cannot choose but remain a closed secret to mankind at large. If, however, it is to become a free gift of Nature like the sun, the air and the water, then it must make itself accessible through a technique which places it within the reach of all, the child no less than the adult, the weak no less than the strong, the householder no less than the *sanyasin*.

Only a very few men of exceptional physical endurance, long life and an extraordinary capacity for not forgetting the distant goal, can, in our time, pursue Patanjali's Ashtang

Yoga to its logical conclusion, its highest purpose: at-one-ment with the Oversoul or *Brahman*. Furthermore, it is so complex that for the majority of *sadhaks* (aspirants) it is likely to become a maze in which they lose their way and mistake the intermediate goals for the final destination. Human nature is such that in pursuing an arduous course, it often forgets the final end, setting up the means as the goal. And so, while Mantra Yoga, Laya Yoga, Hatha Yoga and especially Raja Yoga carry on Patanjali's tradition in modified forms, there emerge three other major forms that represent a great simplification and specialization: the *Jnana* yogin, the *Karma* yogin, or the *Bhakta,* who no longer need to retire from the world or undergo exacting psycho-physical disciplines. Each approaches the goal from a particular angle and reaches it by sheer purposeful concentration.

In Jnana Yoga, one has to develop the faculty of discrimination, so as to be able to distinguish between *agyan* and *gyan*, i.e., ignorance and true knowledge, thereby dispelling the darkness of ignorance, just as with a lighted candle one may dispel darkness from a dark room. In Bhakti Yoga, one begins with the twin principles of *Bhagat* and *Bhagwant,* or the devotee and the deity, and the devotee gradually loses his little self and sees his deity all pervading. Thus his own self expands so as to embrace the totality, thereby changing the course of hatred, separateness and duality into that of love for, at-one-ment and oneness with all living creatures. In Karma Yoga, one may enter the *Karma Kshetra* or the field of actions, under some impelling force to begin with, but in course of time one learns the value of selfless acts performed for their own sake without any attachment to the fruit. By so doing, one may be able to root out feelings of selfishness, egocentricity, self-aggrandizement and self-love and thereby acquire fellow feelings and love for all, see the reflex of the universe within one's own self and that of one's self in all others, and realize ultimately the principle of the Fatherhood of God and the brotherhood of man.

These are, in the main, the three paths, or rather three aspects of an integrated path of head, heart, and hand, whereby one may achieve the desired end, the union of the soul with the Oversoul. They may for convenience be briefly termed the processes of self-mastery, self-sublimation and self-sacrifice. The objective in each is the same, though in the initial stages each starts from dualistic considerations. It is from dualism that one may take to the path of divine knowledge, or universal love and devotion, or of selfless service to humanity leading ultimately to "Cosmic Consciousness," or awareness of the all-pervading Reality as the basis of all that exists.

> *The target ever remains the same,*
> *Though the archers aiming at it be so many.*
>
> RAJAB

Each individual comes into the world with a background of his own, which fits him for a particular type of yoga. Each one receives the mystic call, as one may be inclined temperamentally. To the reflective philosopher gifted with a logical mind, it comes as —"Leave all else and know me." The spiritual aspirant endowed with an emotional mind gets it as—"Leave all else and lose thyself in my love." A highly practical and active mind gets the call as—"Leave all else and serve me." The three approaches tend to overlap and cannot be wholly separated. Something of the Bhakta and the Karma yogin is present in the true Jnani; something of the Jnani and the Bhakta in the true Karma yogin. The matter is not one of exclusiveness but of dominant tendency, and seeming differences in the approaches are not because of any contradiction inherent in the end state attained, but because men vary greatly in temperament. What is possible for the man of a cultured and refined intelligence is impossible for the unsophisticated peasant, and vice versa. Various rivers may wend through different plains, but they all reach the sea.

VI. THE DRAWBACKS TO KARMA AND JNANA YOGA

IF PATANJALI'S SYSTEM AND ITS DERIVATIVES HAVE CERTAIN SERIOUS DRAWBACKS, IT IS IN QUESTION WHETHER THE THREE OTHER MAJOR FORMS ARE WHOLLY WITHOUT THEM. If for the KARMA yogin freedom lies through detachment and desirelessness, is it possible for him to be completely free? Does he not seek emancipation in following his path, and is this itself not a form of desire? Besides, is it psychologically possible for the human mind to detach itself completely from its normal field of experience without first anchoring itself in another and higher one?

It is a universal characteristic of man that he seeks kinship with something other than himself. This is the law of his life and source of all his great achievements. The child is bound to his toys, and the adult to family and society. As in the case of a child, you may not without harm deprive him of his playthings until he has outgrown them psychologically. Likewise, to expect the *sadhak* (seeker) to give up his social and family attachments without first outgrowing them is to cut at the root of life. It will not bring progress but regression, for the man who undertakes it as an enforced discipline only succeeds in repressing his natural desires. The result is not the enhancement of consciousness but its numbing and atrophy, not detachment but indifference. This differs completely from both "attachment" and "detachment," resembling:

> ...the others as death resembles life, being between two lives—unflowering, between the live and the dead nettle.
>
> T. S. ELIOT

The discipline of Karma Yoga is a necessary one, but if it is to fulfill its spiritual end it must be completed by another discipline of an esoteric kind, without which it tends to reduce itself to an ineffectual attempt to lift oneself up by one's shoestrings. As for the Jnana yogin, Jnana may carry him very far indeed. It may take him beyond the gross physical plane into the spiritual ones. But can knowledge carry him beyond itself?

Jnana forms one of the *koshas*, or sheaths, that surround the soul, and thus is both a help and a hindrance. It has indubitably the power to rid the soul of all encumbrances grosser than itself, but having reached thus far it tends to prevent further progress. And since it is not of the true essence of the soul, the Absolute, it cannot be wholly above the realm of *Kala* or Time.

Mystics distinguish between the two realms of time, *Kala* and *Mahakala,* thus: the first of these extends over the physical world and the less gross regions immediately above it, whereas the second stretches to all the higher planes that are not of pure spirit. Hence, the gains that the jnani achieves may be out of the reach of time as we normally conceive it (*kala*), but they are not wholly beyond the reach of greater time (*mahakala*). It need hardly be pointed out that what is true of Jnana Yoga is also true of those derivative forms of yoga that depend upon the pranic energies, Kundalini Yoga, Hatha Yoga, etc. They, too, are not of the true nature of the Atman, and as such cannot lead It to a state beyond the realm of relativity.

Besides its inability to ensure absolute freedom, Jnana Yoga is not a path accessible to the average man. It demands extraordinary intellectual powers and stamina which few possess. It was to meet this difficulty as well as that posed by Karma Yoga when practiced by itself, that Bhakti Yoga came into prominence.

VII. THE LIMITATION OF BHAKTI YOGA

HE WHO NORMALLY WOULD NOT BE ABLE TO DETACH HIMSELF FROM THE WORLD NOR HAD THE MENTAL POWERS TO ANALYZE THE TRUE SELF FROM THE UNTRUE COULD BY THE POWER OF LOVE LEAP OR BRIDGE THE GAP AND REACH THE GOAL. But how can man love that which has neither form nor shape? So the bhakta anchors himself in the love of some *Isht-deva,* some definite manifestation of God. Yet in overcoming this practical difficulty he exposes himself to the same limitations as the jnani. The chosen Isht-deva by its very nature represents a limitation upon the Nameless and Formless Absolute. And even if the Bhakta reaches the level of that manifestation, can that limited being take him beyond itself to that which has no limitation? The experience of Sri Ramakrishna (1836-1880) in our own time brings out this limitation. He had always been a worshiper of the Divine Mother and she often blessed him with her visions. But he always perceived her as something other than himself, as a power outside himself and one for whose operation he could often become a medium, but in which he could not merge himself. When he subsequently met Totapuri, a realized soul, he saw that he must get beyond this stage to one where there was no name or form and where the Self and the Overself became one. When he attempted to enter into such a state he discovered that his earlier attainments became a hurdle in spite of all his efforts. He tells us:

> I could not cross the realm of name and form and bring my mind to the unconditioned state. I had no difficulty in withdrawing my mind from all objects except one, and this was the all too familiar form of the Blissful Mother—radiant and of the essence of pure consciousness—which appeared before me as a living reality and would not allow me to pass the realm of name and form.

Again and again I tried to concentrate my mind upon the Advaita teachings, but every time the Mother's form stood in my way. In despair I said to "the naked one" (his Master Totapuri), "It is hopeless. I cannot raise my mind to the unconditioned state and come face to face with the Atman." He grew excited and sharply said, "What! You can't do it? But you have to." He cast his eyes around for something and finding a piece of glass he took it up and pressing its point between my eyebrows said, "Concentrate your mind on this point." Then with stern determination I again sat to meditate, and as soon as the gracious form of the Divine Mother appeared before me, I used my discrimination as a sword and with it severed it into two. There remained no more obstruction to my mind, which at once soared beyond the relative plane, and I lost myself in Samadhi.*

It is clear therefore that while the bhakta can go very far spiritually, can greatly enhance his consciousness, gain miraculous powers, and anchored in a higher love rise above the love of this world, it is nevertheless not possible for him to get beyond the plane of "name and form," and therefore of relativity. He may get lost in the contemplation of the Godhead with His amazing attributes, but he cannot experience the same in its *Nirguna* and its *Anami,* its "Unconditioned" and "Nameless" state. He can feel himself saturated with Cosmic Conciousness, but it comes to him as something outside himself as a gift of grace, and he is not able to lose himself in It and become one with the Ocean of Being. If he does seek to attain that state, his accomplishment as a Bhakta, instead of helping him further, tends to hinder and obstruct him.

The two things that emerge from an examination of the popular forms of yoga that were evolved after Patanjali are: first that the soul can rise above physical consciousness, given means whereby it can focus its energies, and second that full

---

*Sayings of Sri Ramakrishna (Mylapore-Madras, 1954), page 313.

spiritual realization or true samadhi is not merely a matter of transcending the physical (though that is necessary as a first step), but is the end of a complex inner journey in which there are many intermediate stages the attainment of which, under certain conditions, may be mistaken for the final goal and may thus debar further progress. The problem that arises before the true seeker in the face of such a situation is to discover a means other than that of pranas, jnana, or bhakti of an Isht-deva, as not only to enable the spirit-currents to be released from their present physical bondage, but also to enable the soul to be drawn upward unhindered from one spiritual plane to another until it transcends completely all the realms of relativity of *naam* and *rup,* of *kala* and *mahakala,* and reaches its goal: at-one-ment with the Nameless and Formless One.

PART 2
SURAT SHABD YOGA

I. SCRIPTURAL REFERENCES

IT IS IN THE CONTEXT OF THE LIMITATIONS OF THE OTHER YOGAS IN REACHING THE NAMELESS STATE THAT SURAT SHABD YOGA, OR THE YOGA OF THE CELESTIAL SOUND CURRENT, ASSUMES ITS UNIQUE IMPORTANCE. Those who have mastered this yoga teach that the Absolute projects itself into form and assumes two primary attributes: Light and Sound. It is no mere accident, they point out, that in the revelatory literature of all major religions there are frequent references to the "Word" which occupies a central position in their pattern. In the Gospels we have:

> *In the beginning was the Word and the Word*
> *was with God and the Word was God.*

ST. JOHN

In ancient Indian scriptures we read repeatedly of *Aum*, the sacred Word pervading the three realms of *bhur*, *bhuva* and *swah* (i.e., the physical, astral and causal).

> *The earth and sky are of naught but Shabd (Word).*
> *From Shabd alone the light was born,*
> *From Shabd alone creation came,*
> *Shabd is the essential core in all.*

NANAK

> *Shabd is the directive agent of God, the cause of all creation.*
>
> PRABHATI

The Muslim Sufis declare:

> *Creation came into being from Saut (Sound or Word) and from Saut spread all light.*
>
> SHAMAS TABREZ

> *The Great Name is the very essence and life of all names and forms.*
> *Its manifest form sustains creation;*
> *It is the great ocean of which we are merely the waves,*
> *He alone can comprehend this who has mastered our discipline.*
>
> ABDUL RAZAQ KASHI

Moses heard the commandments of God amidst thunder and flame, while in Zoroastrian and Taoist thought alike there are references to the "Creative Verbum," the "Divine Light," and to the "Wordless Word," the silent Word.

Some learned scholars and theologians in subsequent times, because of their own limited experience, have interpreted these descriptions as metaphoric references to intuitive or intellectual enlightenment. On closer examination such a position will be found to be untenable. The terms "Word" or *Logos* as used by the Greeks, Hebrews and Europeans, may be distorted to mean "reason" or "order," and "light," may even be made to mean no more than mental illumination, but their equivalents in other religious literature —*nad, udgit, akash-bani, shabd, naam, saut, bang-i-Ilahi, nida-i-asmani, sraosha, tao,* and *jyoti, prakash, tajalli, nur-i-yazdani,* etc., refuse to bear such a travesty of their original mystic meaning. What is more, some seers have stated their real connotation in such a way that there can be no scope for equivocation or room for doubt that what is involved is not figurative expression of ordinary mental experience, but transcendent inner perception. Thus, in the Revelation of St. John we have:

His eyes were as a flame of fire...His voice as the sound of many waters...His countenance was as the sun shineth in his strength...
And I heard a Voice from heaven, as the voice of many waters, and as the voice of a great thunder: and I heard the voice of harpers, harping with their harps.

While in the Upanishads we are told:

First the murmuring sounds resembling those of the waves of the ocean, the fall of rain and then running rivulets, after which the bhervi will be heard, intermingled with the sounds of bell and conch.

NAD BIND UPANISHAD

The Prophet Mohammed heard celestial music which gradually assumed the shape of Gabriel and formed itself into words; while Baha U'llah relates:

Myriads of mystic tongues find utterance in one speech, and myriads of His hidden mysteries are revealed in a single melody; yet alas, there is no ear to hear nor heart to understand!
Blind thine eyes, that thou mayest behold My Beauty, and stop thine ears that thou mayest hearken unto the sweet melody of My Voice.

II. THE SHABD OR WORD

REFERENCES TO LIGHT AND SOUND, SAY THE MASTERS OF SURAT SHABD YOGA, ARE NOT FIGURATIVE BUT LITERAL, REFERRING NOT TO THE OUTER ILLUMINATIONS OR SOUNDS OF THIS WORLD, BUT TO INNER TRANSCENDENT ONES. They teach that the transcendent Sound and Light are the primal manifestations of God when He projects Himself into creation. In His Nameless state He is neither light nor darkness, neither sound nor silence, but when He assumes shape and form, Light and Sound emerge as His primary attributes.

This spirit force, Word, *Naam*, *Kalma* or God-in-action, is responsible for all that is, and the physical universes that we know are not the only ones that It has created. It has brought into being myriad regions and myriad creations over and above the physical. Indeed the whole is a grand unfathomable illimitable pattern in which the Positive pole (*Sach Khand* or *Sat Lok*) is a plane of pure, unalloyed spirit, while the Negative pole (*Pind*) is of gross physical matter with which we in this world are familiar. In between are countless regions which they who have journeyed from one end to the other often divide into three distinct planes in accordance with the balance of Positive or spiritual and Negative or material forces in each plane.

The Masters teach that the one constant principle that links all these planes from pure spirit to gross matter is the principle of the flaming sound or the sounding flame. The Word or *Shabd* as it descends downward assumes a varying density of spirituo-material forces. Mystics speak of the purple light and the light of the noonday or setting sun, and refer to the sounds of flutes, harps, violins, conches, thunder, bells, running water, etc., but though manifesting differently at different levels the *Shabd* yet remains constant in Itself.

As a river springing from the snowy peak of a towering mountain flows toward the sea, it undergoes many changes of setting, shape, motion and appearance, and yet its waters remain the same.

If one could discover this audible life-stream within oneself, if one could discover its lower reaches, one could use it as a pathway leading inevitably to its source. The currents might at certain points enter gorges and rapids, but nevertheless they are the surest way on the upward journey. Be a range howsoever unscalable, the waters will have cut a pass and carved a passage, and he who will avail himself of their guidance would never fail to find a way. And since this *Naam* or Word-current springs from the *Anaam* or the Wordless, he who holds firmly to It will inevitably reach the starting point, transcending plane after plane of varying relativity until he arrives at the very source of name and form; thence to merge into That which has no name or form.

III. THE EASY WAY: COMPARISONS AND DIFFICULTIES

NOT ONLY DO THOSE FOLLOWING THIS PATH REACH THE ULTIMATE END, BUT THEY DO SO WITH GREATER ECONOMY OF EFFORT THAN IS POSSIBLE BY THE OTHER METHODS. It begins at the point where other yogas normally tend to end. Sahasrar, the region of the thousand-petaled lights, which marks the end of the normal yogin's journey after traversing the various bodily *chakras* (psycho-physical centers) is well-nigh the first step to be taken by the follower of the Surat Shabd Yoga.

That this should be so is not a mere chance or accident, for the fact is that the Surat Shabd Yoga adopts a more scientific and natural approach to man's spiritual problems. Why, it asserts, if the spiritual current reaches the bodily chakras not from below but from above, should it be necessary to master each of these chakras in turn? A man standing at the heart of a valley, if he wishes to reach the river's source, does not have to travel down to its mouth and then retraverse the distance. It further holds that if prana and mind (even at their most refined) are not of the true essence of the spirit, then how can they be the best means of disengaging it from its encrustations? If it could be put in touch with that which is of its own essential nature, like would draw like, and with the minimum of effort the desired end would be achieved. It is from the point of the *tisra-til,* the third eye, that the spiritual current spreads itself into the body. All that is needed is to check its downward flow at this point by controlling one's senses and it would, of its own accord, collect itself and flow backwards toward its source.

Further, by refusing to disturb the pranic or kundalinic energies, this yoga greatly reduces the strain of physical transcendence. By contacting the Sound-principle, the sensory currents are automatically drawn upward without the practitioner consciously striving to achieve this end, and the motor currents are left untouched. Not only does this simplify the process of entry into the state of samadhi, but that of returning from it as well. The adept in this path needs no outer assistance for coming back into physical consciousness, as is the case with some other yogic forms; spiritual ascension and descent are entirely voluntary and can be achieved by him with the rapidity of thought.

It is this simplicity of approach coupled with economy of effort that has induced many to call the Surat Shabd Yoga the *Sehaj Marg* or the Easy Way. It is this same quality of *sehaj*, of naturalness and ease, that also makes the Surat Shabd Yoga accessible to all. The music of the Divine Word is vibrating in all alike, and he who follows Its path, needs no special requirements, whether physical or intellectual. It is as much open to the old as to the young, to the sinners as to the saints, to the simple as to the learned, to women and children as to men. Indeed, women and children and the unsophisticated, owing to their simpler modes of thought and their spontaneous faith, often make quicker initial headway with this method than their more sophisticated brethren. As no rigorous and extensive disciplines of food, physical exercises, etc., are required, it does not necessitate *sanyasa* or complete renunciation of the world, and is as much open to the *grehastis*, the married, as to the *brahmcharis*, those who are under a vow of celibacy.

However, to say that the Surat Shabd Yoga is the most perfect of the yogic sciences and the most natural, and the most accessible, is not to say that it demands no effort and that anyone can just take to it and succeed. The fact is that competent teachers of this crown of all sciences are rare and that even when a teacher is found, few are prepared to undergo the kind of discipline required.

Since the stress in this yoga is always on the inner, never on the outer, no path could in a way be more exacting for the general run of humanity. Many can spend whole lives in outer ritual and ceremonial but few can attain perfect inner concentration, undisturbed by mundane thoughts, even for a few moments. Further, most men are so deeply engrossed with the love of the world that even after having had a glimpse of inner treasures they are reluctant to give up their worldly ways and concentrate on the possession of that which makes one the master of all. Hence it was that Kabir compared it to walking on a naked sword, while the Sufis spoke of it as the *rah-i-mustqim*, finer than a hair and sharper than the razor's edge. Christ described it as the "strait and narrow way" that only a few ever tread. But for one whom the world lures not and who is filled with a passionate love of God, nothing could be easier and quicker. He needs no other force than that of his own urge and, purified of earthly attachments by his sincere and strong longing, his soul shall wing homeward, borne on the stream of Shabd toward its point of origin, the haven of bliss and peace.

IV. THE LIVING MASTER

APART FROM ITS SCIENTIFIC APPROACH, ITS COMPARATIVELY EASY ACCESSIBILITY, ITS QUALITY OF NATURALNESS AND ITS FREEDOM FROM THE DRAWBACKS OF OTHER YOGIC FORMS, ANOTHER DISTINCTIVE FEATURE OF THE YOGA OF THE SOUND CURRENT IS THE UNIQUE AND PERVASIVE EMPHASIS IT LAYS ON THE NEED AT EVERY STEP FOR A SATGURU, *PIR-E-RAH* OR *MURSHID-I-KAMIL* (A COMPETENT, LIVING MASTER). The *Guru-shish* or *Guru-sikh* relationship is important in all forms of practical yoga, but it is pivotal here in a unique sense. For the Guru in the Surat Shabd Yoga is not only a being who explains to us the real nature of existence, instructs us in the true values of life and tells us of the *sadhnas* (spiritual practices) to be practiced for inner attainment, he is all this and more. He is the inner guide as well, leading the soul from plane to plane to its ultimate destination, a guide without whose aid the soul would mistake the intermediate stages for the final goal and would encounter barriers which it would be unable to surmount.

> *Find a Master spirit, for without his active help and guidance, this journey is beset with dangers, perils and fears.*
>
> JALALUD-DIN RUMI

The Master is indeed the "Intercessor" or *Rasul*, who moves between man and God;

> *No man cometh unto the Father but by me.*
>
> ST. JOHN

> *No man knoweth who the Father is, but the Son; and he to whom the Son will reveal Him.*
>
> ST. LUKE AND ST. MATTHEW

The role of the Master being what it is, it is little wonder that all mystics who have pursued this way should have sung of him with superlative reverence and adoration. From Kabir, we read:

> *I wish and long for the dust of his feet—the dust that has created the universe;*
> *His lotus feet are the true wealth and a haven of peace.*
> *They grant ineffable wisdom and lead one on the path Godward.*

And the Sikh scriptures sing:

> *Sweet are the lotus feet of the Master;*
> *With God's writ one sees them;*
> *And myriad are the blessings that follow upon such a vision.*
>
> GURU ARJAN

From the Sufis, we have:

> *If I were to sing praises of his countless blessings till eternity,*
> *I could hardly say anything of them.*
>
> JALALUD-DIN RUMI

Some mystics even go to the extent of raising his position above that of God:

> *The Master is greater than God.*
>
> KABIR

> *The Guru and God both stand manifested, whom may I adore and render obeisance?*
> *Wonderful indeed is the Guru who has revealed the God-power within.*
>
> SEHJO BAI

> *When I churned the sea of body, a strange truth came to light,*
> *God was identified in the Master and no distinction could Nanak find.*
>
> GURU RAM DAS

THE LIVING MASTER

All this may lead one to suspect human idolatry. He may ask: "Why this deification of a human being? Why such praise heaped upon one who is mortal?" Mystics at times have responded to this question with indifference:

> *Enter within and verify for yourself,*
> *Who is greater of the two: God or the Guru.*
>
> GURBANI

> *People decry that Khusro has turned idolator;*
> *Indeed I have, but what has the world to do with me?*
>
> AMIR KHUSRO

But sometimes, they have answered directly:

> *Without the munificence of the Master one gets naught,*
> *Even if one engages in a million meritorious deeds.*
>
> GURBANI

> *Devotion to God keeps one entangled in this (physical) life—just consider gravely,*
> *But devotion to the Master carries one back unto God.*
>
> KABIR

> *God drove me into the wilderness of the world, but the Master has snapped for me the ceaseless chain of transmigration.*
>
> SEHJO BAI

V. RECOGNIZING A LIVING MASTER

WHERE THE GUIDANCE OF A COMPETENT LIVING MASTER IS SUCH A PRIME NECESSITY, THE TASK OF FINDING AND RECOGNIZING SUCH A GENUINE SOUL ASSUMES PARAMOUNT IMPORTANCE. There is no dearth of false prophets and of wolves in sheep's clothing. The very term *Satguru,* or true Master, implies the existence of its opposite, and it is the false that meet our gaze at every turn. However difficult it may be to find a God-man (for such beings are rare, unobtrusive in their humility and reluctant to declare themselves by spectacular miracles or court the public limelight), it is nevertheless not impossible to single him out from the rest. He is a living embodiment of what he teaches, and though appearing poor, he is rich in his poverty:

> *We may seem beggars, but our actions are more than royal.*
>
> SHAMAS TABREZ

He gives his teachings and instructions as a free gift of nature, never seeking anything in return, maintaining himself by his own labors and never living on the offerings of others:

> *Bow not before one who calls himself a Master, yet lives on the charity of others.*
> *He alone is of the true path who earns his own livelihood and befriends the needy.*
>
> GURU RAM DAS

Further, a genuine Master-soul never sets up any contradictions in our minds; all the distinctions between faith and faith, creed and creed, vanish at his touch, and the unity of inner experience embodied in the various scriptures stands clearly revealed:

> *It is only the jeweller's eye that at a glance can tell the ruby.*
>
> BHAI NAND LAL

The one recurrent theme of such a Master's teaching is that in spite of all the outward distinctions that confuse and confound us, the inner spiritual essence of all religious teachings is the same. Hence the Masters come not to propagate new creeds or dogmas but to fulfill the existing Law:

> *O Nanak, know him to be a perfect Master who unites all in one fold.*
>
> GURU NANAK

Thus it is the inner message that is ever paramount in the teachings of a real Master. He can best interpret the true import of the scriptures, but he speaks not as one who is learned in such matters, but as one who has himself experienced what such writings record. He may use the scriptures to convince his listeners that what he teaches is the most ancient truth, yet he himself is never subject to them and his message moves above the merely intellectual level—it is inspired by the vividness and intensity of direct first-hand experience. "How can we agree," said Kabir to the scholars and pandits, "when I speak from inner experience and you only from bookish learning."

A true Master makes the seeker turn always inward, telling him of the rich treasures within:

> *Dost thou reckon thyself a puny form,*
> *When within thee the Universe is folded?*
>
> ALI

> *The kingdom of God cometh not with observation,*
> *The kingdom of God is within you.*
>
> ST. LUKE

Thus the spiritual practices enjoined by a perfect teacher will focus on transcendental hearing and seeing accompanied by a steady outer purification of one's thoughts and deeds by means of moderation and introspective self-criticism, rather than by torture, austerity, asceticism, or other such extreme practices. A true Master always insists on the maintaining of a record of daily lapses in thought, word and deed, from non-injury, truth, chastity, universal love and selfless service of all, the five cardinal virtues that pave the way for spirituality.

Yet the most important and least fallible sign of the *Satguru* is that his teachings will always be centered on this inner sicence, and at the time of initiation, or acceptance of a seeker as a disciple, he will be able to give the disciple a definite experience—be it ever so rudimentary—of the Light and Sound within and, when the disciple has learned to rise above body-consciousness, his Radiant Form will appear unsought to guide him onward on the long journey.

> *The wondrous and luminous form of the Master only a true Master can make manifest to the spirit.*
> GURU NANAK

He is a Guru in vain who cannot turn the darkness (*gu*) into light (*ruh*). If he is a genuine teacher, he will never promise salvation that comes only after death. Accordingly, to him it is always a matter of now and here. One who has not attained liberation in life, cannot hope to achieve it after death. A Master will further maintain that spirituality is a science, albeit a subjective one, and that every individual can and must verify its truth in the laboratory of his own body, provided he can create the requisite condition, which is one-pointed concentration.

VI. SADACHAR: CHARITY

IT IS THE NECESSITY FOR SELF-DISCIPLINE THAT MAKES *SADACHAR* THE SECOND CONDITION, AFTER FINDING A LIVING MASTER, THAT MUST BE FULFILLED BEFORE SUCCESS IN THIS TRUEST OF ALL YOGAS CAN BE ATTAINED. The word *sadachar* is not easy to translate. One can find many literal equivalents, but none of them really express its extensive and many-sided significance. In brief, it stands for the good and pure life. It does not imply any rigid code or set moral formulae, but suggests purity and simplicity, which radiate from within and spread outwards, permeating every action, every word, every thought. It is as much concerned with one's personal habits, good and hygienic, as with one's individual and social ethics. And on its ethical side, it is concerned not merely with one's relation to one's fellow men but to all living things, i.e., harmony which is the result of recognition that all things are from the same Essence, and so a worm is as much a part of Brahman as the mightiest of gods, Indra.

The first lesson taught by a true Guru is that of "the identity of substance," and he who has grasped this truth will discipline his life accordingly. His would be a life of detachment or of *nishkama*. But detachment would not be for him a life of indifference or of ascetic renunciation. To know all life is to discover a new bond between oneself and the rest of creation. He who knows this cannot be merely "indifferent." He must perforce be filled to overflowing with sympathy for all that he confronts, and sympathy toward the whole must imply a certain holy indifference to the part. He will no longer be tied to his own narrow individual interests, but will share his love and resources with all. He will develop, slowly but surely, something of the compassion of the Buddha and the love of Christ. Nor will he feel himself called upon to leave the world for the solitude of the forest, the mountain or the desert cave.

The detachment must be an inner one, and one who cannot achieve it at home will not achieve it in the forest. He will recognize the great use of occasional retreats from worldly affairs and cares to the silence of solitary meditation and concentration, but he will not seek to escape from life and its responsibilities. He will be a loving husband and a good father, but while being these he will never forget the ultimate purpose of life, always knowing how to give unto Caesar that which is Caesar's, and preserving for God that which is God's. To him, *sanyasa* (renunciation) is not a matter of outer evasion or escapism but of inner freedom:

> *Let contentment be your ear-rings,*
> *And endeavor for the Divine and respect for the higher Self your wallet,*
> *And constant meditation on Him your ashes,*
> *Let preparedness for death be your cloak,*
> *And let your body be like unto a chaste virgin.*
> *Let your Master's teachings be your supporting staff.*

JAP JI

The two cardinal virtues that such a man will cultivate will be charity and chastity. He will be large of heart and bounteous, caring more for the sufferings of others than for his own, and easily forgiving those that injure him. He will be simple and restrained in his habits. His wants will be few and easily satisifed, for one who has too many desires and too many attachments cannot be pure of heart. For him chastity will extend even to giving up meat and drink. When all life is one, to live upon the flesh of other living beings would be to defile oneself. And when one's goal is to attain even higher realms of consciousness, to resort to narcotics and intoxicants is only to court regression.

> *Truth is above all*
> *Yet higher still is true living.*

SRI RAG

SADACHAR: CHARITY 45

VII. SADACHAR: CHASTITY

IT IS NOT AN IDIOSYNCRACY OF INDIAN SEERS THAT THEY SHOULD HAVE MADE ABSTINENCE FROM MEAT AND DRINK A NECESSARY PART OF THE SPIRITUAL DISCIPLINE. We find similar injunctions in the Holy Bible:

> *Be not among winebibbers; among riotous eaters of flesh.*
>
> PROVERBS 23:20

> *It is good neither to eat flesh, nor to drink wine, nor anything whereby thy brother stumbleth, or is offended, or is made weak.*
>
> ROMANS 14:21

> *Meats for the belly, and belly for meats; but God shall destroy both it and them. Now the body is not for fornication but for the Lord; and the Lord for the body.*
>
> CORINTHIANS 6:13

In the *Essene Gospel of John* (direct translation from the Aramaic of the pure original words of Jesus), it is written:

> But they answered Him: "Whither should we go, Master, . . . for with you are the words of eternal life. Tell us, what are the sins we must shun, that we may nevermore see disease?"
>
> Jesus answered: "Be it so according to your faith," and He sat down among them, saying:
>
> "It was said to them of olden time, 'Honor thy Heavenly Father and thy Earthly Mother, and their commandments, that thy days may be long upon the earth.' And next was given this commandment: 'Thou shalt not kill,' for life is given to all by God, and that which God has given, let not man take

away. For I tell you truly, from one Mother proceeds all that lives upon the earth. Therefore he who kills, kills his brother. And from him will the Earthly Mother turn away, and will pluck from him her quickening breasts. And he will be shunned by her angels, and Satan will have his dwelling in his body. And the flesh of slain beasts in his body will become his own tomb. For I tell you truly, he who kills, kills himself, and whosoever eats the flesh of slain beasts, eats of the body of death. And their death will become his death. For the wages of sin is death. Kill not, neither eat the flesh of your innocent prey, lest you become the slaves of Satan. For that is the path of sufferings, and it leads unto death. But do the Will of God, that his angels may serve you on the way of life. Obey, therefore, the words of God: 'Behold, I have given you every herb, bearing seed, which is upon the face of all the earth, and every tree, in which is the fruit of a tree yielding seed; to you it shall be for meat. And to every beast of the earth, and to every fowl of the air, and to everything that creepeth upon the earth wherein there is breath of life, I give every green herb for meat.' Also the milk of everything that moveth and that liveth upon each shall be meat for you; even as the green herb have I given unto them, so I give their milk unto you. But flesh, and the blood which quickens it, shall ye not eat.''

And Jesus continued: "God commanded your forefathers, 'Thou shalt not kill.' But their heart was hardened and they killed. Then Moses desired that at least they should not kill men, and he suffered them to kill beasts. And then the heart of your forefathers was hardened yet more, and they killed men and beasts likewise. But I say to you: Kill neither men, nor beasts, nor yet the food which goes into your mouth. For if you eat living food the same will quicken you, but if you kill your food, the dead food will kill you also. For life comes only from life, and from death comes always death. For everything which kills your foods, kills your bodies also. And everything which kills your bodies, kills your souls also. And your bodies become what your foods are, even as your spirits, likewise, become what your thoughts are.'"*

With the chastity in food and drink will go another kind of chastity, the one that pertains to sex. One will not suppress all sexual desire, for repression can only breed neurosis and prepare the way for a downfall, but he will be ever seeking to sublimate it. He will understand that nature's purpose in this instinct is to preserve the race and will channel it so as to fulfill that purpose, never making it an end in itself, a source of physical pleasure, for when it becomes that, it turns into a drug that anaesthetizes the spirit.

In short, the sincere and conscientious aspirant will reorient his entire mode of life, in eating and drinking, thinking, acting, feeling, etc. He will gradually weed out of his mind all irrelevant and unhealthy desires, until he gradually attains the state of purity and simplicity that marks the child.

> *Verily I say unto you, except ye be converted and become as little children, ye shall not enter into the Kingdom of God.*
>
> ST. MATTHEW

Through all this process of reintegration, his inspiration will be the example of his Master whose life will be a living testament beckoning him toward the ideal of sadachar, and the experience he has of the Word within will stand as a proof of the truth of what his Master teaches. Sadachar is no dry discipline that can be attained by following certain set formulae. It is a way of life, and in such matters only heart to heart can speak. It is this that makes *Satsang,* or association with a true Master, so

---

*Szekeley, Edmond Bordeaux, trans, *The Essene Gospel of Peace* (San Diego, 1975) pp 43-49.

important. It not only serves as a constant reminder of the goal before the seeker, but through the magic touch of personal contact, gradually transforms his entire mode of thinking and feeling. As his heart and mind under this benign influence grow gradually purer, his life more fully centers in the divine. In short, as he increasingly realizes in practice the ideal of sadachar, his thoughts, now scattered and dissipated, will gain equipoise and integration till they arrive at so fine a focus that the veils of inner darkness are burnt to cinders and the inner glory stands revealed.

VIII. SADHNA: SPIRITUAL DISCIPLINE

ALL THE GREAT TEACHERS OF HUMANITY, AT ALL TIMES AND IN ALL CLIMES—THE VEDIC RISHIS, ZOROASTER, MAHAVIRA, BUDDHA, CHRIST, MOHAMMED, NANAK, KABIR, BABA FARID, HAZRAT BAHU, SHAMAS TABREZ, MAULANA RUMI, TULSI SAHIB, SWAMIJI AND MANY OTHERS—GAVE TO THE WORLD BUT ONE *SADHNA* OR SPIRITUAL DISCIPLINE. As God is one, the God-way too cannot but be one. The true religion or the way back to God is of God's own making. It is only the spirit—disencumbered and depersonalized—that can undertake the spiritual journey. The inner man, the soul in man, has to rise above body-consciousness before it can traverse into higher consciousness or the consciousness of the cosmos and of the beyond. The seat of the soul is between and behind the eyebrows. This is accepted by all yogas. It is to this point that mystics refer when they speak of *shiv netra, divya chakshu, tisra til, Brahm-rendra, triambka, trilochana, nukta-i-sweda, koh-i-toor,* third eye, single eye, figuratively called the still point, the mount of transfiguration, etc. It is at this point that the sadhak having closed his eyes must focus his attention, but the effort at concentration must be an effortless one and there must be no question of any physical or mental strain.

In actual practice of the sadhna, which is the third condition for succeeding in the science of Surat Shabd Yoga, stress is laid on *Simran*, *Dhyan* and *Bhajan*, each of which plays a specific role in unfoldment of the Self. The Master gives *Simran* or mental repetition of charged words, which help in gathering together the wandering wits of the practitioner to the still point, to which place the sensory currents now pervading from top to toe are withdrawn, and one becomes lost to the consciousness of the flesh.

The successful completion of this process of itself leads to *Dhyan* or concentration. Dhyan is derived from the Sanskrit root *dhi*, meaning "to bind" and "to hold on." With the inner eye opened, the aspirant now sees shimmering streaks of heaven's light within him and this keeps his attention anchored. Gradually, the light grows steady in his sadhna, for it works as a sheet-anchor for the soul. In turn Dhyan, when perfected, leads one to *Bhajan* or attuning to the music which emerges from within the center of the holy light. This enchanting holy melody has a magnetic pull which is irresistible, and the soul cannot but follow it to the spiritual source from whence the music emerges.

> *Within thee is Light and within the Light*
>   *the Sound*
> *And the same shall keep thee attached*
>   *to the True One.*
>
> GURBANI

The soul is helped by the triple process to slide out of the shackles of the body and becomes anchored in the heavenly radiance of its Atman Self and is led on to the heavenly home of the Father. Having reached the journey's end, the seeker too merges with the Word and enters the company of the Free Ones. He may continue to live like other men in this world of human beings, but his spirit knows no limitations and is as infinite as God Himself. The wheel of transmigration can no longer affect him, and his consciousness knows no restrictions. Like his Master before him, he has become a Conscious Co-worker of the Divine Plan. He does nothing for himself but works in God's name. Like a flower shedding fragrance, he spreads the message of freedom wherever he goes.

> *Those who have communed with the Word,*
>   *their toils shall end.*
> *And their faces shall flame with glory.*
> *Not only shall they have salvation,*
> *O Nanak, but many more shall find freedom*
>   *with them.*

JAP JI

IX. THE RADIANT FORM OF THE MASTER

WHEN STUDENTS OF THE OTHER FORMS OF YOGA REACH THE STATE OF FULL PHYSICAL TRANSCENDENCE AFTER A LONG AND EXACTING MASTERY OF THE LOWER CHAKRAS, THEY GENERALLY ASSUME THAT THEY HAVE REACHED THE JOURNEY'S END. The inner plane at which they find themselves—the realm of Sahasrar or Sahasdal Kamal, often symbolized by the sun-wheel, the lotus or the multifoliate rose—is indeed incomparably more beautiful than anything on earth, and in comparison appears timeless. But when the student of the Surat Shabd Yoga succeeds in rising above physical consciousness, he finds the Radiant Form of his Master waiting unsought to receive him. Indeed, it is at this point that the real *Guru-shishya* or teacher-student relationship is established. Up to this stage, the Guru had been little more than a human teacher, but now he is seen as the divine guide or *Gurudev,* who shows the inner way:

> *The feet of my Master have been manifested in*
>   *my forehead,*
> *And all my wanderings and tribulations have*
>   *ended.*
>
> GURU ARJAN
>
> *With the appearance of the Radiant Form of the*
> *Master within,*
> *No secret remains hidden in the womb of time.*

Christ also speaks in the same strain:

> *There is nothing covered, that shall not be*
> *revealed, and hid, that shall not be known.*
>
> ST. MATTHEW

Under the guidance of this Celestial Guide the soul learns to overcome the first shock of joy, and realizes that its goal lies still far ahead. Accompanied by the Radiant Form and drawn by the Audible Life Current, it traverses from region to region, from plane to plane, dropping off kosha after kosha, until at last it stands wholly divested of all that is not of its nature. Should the soul confront any obstacles on its homing flight, its Radiant Friend is always beside it to lead it past and protect it from all pitfalls.

The road through the higher planes lies charted before the soul as completely as that for Hatha yogins of the lower bodily chakras, and with such a Power to bear it, and such a Friend to guide, nothing can deter or entrap, nothing can disturb the steadiness of its course. "Take hold of the garment, O brave soul, of One who knows well all places, physical, mental, supra-mental and spiritual, for he will remain thy friend in life as well as in death, in this world and the worlds beyond," exhorted Jalalud-din Rumi.

Chance winds may blow others apart and death may come to part the most faithful lovers; he alone is unfailing in life as well as in death:

*I have commanded you; and, lo! I am with you
always, even unto the end of the world.*
ST. MATTHEW

*He alone is a friend who accompanies me on my
last journey,
And shields me before the judgment seat of God.*
GURBANI

The true Guru-shish relationship has very often been described:

*Who is the true Guru for a disciple?
Shabd indeed is the Guru and Surat the disciple
of the Dhun (Sound).*
GURU NANAK

The Word was made flesh, and dwelt among us.
ST. JOHN

*The Word of the Master is Master indeed, full of
life-giving water,
He who follows His Word doth verily cross the
strands of time.*
GURU RAM DAS

*The disciple-Surat can traverse the Path only
with the Shabd-Guru,
Exploring the heavenly mysteries, it doth find
rest in the inverted well (of the head).*
TULSI SAHIB

*Know it for certain that Shabd-Guru is the
veritable Guru,
Surat can truly become the disciple of the Dhun
by being a Gur-mukh (receptacle for the Word).*
BHAI GURDAS

*Guru resides in the gagan (spiritual realm above)
and the disciple in the ghat (between the
two eyebrows).
When the two, the Surat and the Shabd, do
meet, they get united eternally.*
KABIR

THE RADIANT FORM OF THE MASTER

X. LOVE AND THE LOVER'S RELATIONSHIP

ON THIS MYSTIC PATH REASONING IS THE HELP, BUT REASONING IS ALSO THE HINDRANCE. LOVE ALONE CAN BRIDGE THE GULF, SPAN THE CHASM, AND KNIT THE FINITE TO THE INFINITE, THE MORTAL TO THE IMMORTAL, THE RELATIVE TO THE ABSOLUTE. It alone is the key to the inner kingdom:

> *He that loveth not knoweth not God, for God is love.*
>
> ST. JOHN

> *The secret of God's mysteries is love.*
>
> RUMI

> *By love may He be gotten and holden, but by thought never.*
>
> THE CLOUD OF UNKNOWING

> *Verily, verily I say unto thee, that only they that have loved have reached the Lord.*
>
> GOBIND SINGH

> *The world is lost in reading scriptures, yet never comes to knowledge,*
> *But one who knows a jot of love, to him all is revealed.*
>
> KABIR

Such love is not of this world or of this flesh. It is the call of soul unto soul, of like unto like, the purgatory and the paradise.

> *Speak not of Leila's or of Majnun's woe*
> *Thy love hath put to naught the loves of long ago.*
>
> SAADI

> *Live free of love for its very peace is anguish.*
>
> ARABIAN POEM

A million speak of love, yet how few know,
True love is not to lose remembrance even for an instant.

KABIR

Indeed, it is the quality of ceaseless remembrance of the Beloved that is of the essence of love. He who remembers in such fashion lives in perpetual obedience to his Beloved's commandments and burns in its fire the dross of the ego.

If thou wouldst journey on the road of love,
First learn to humble thyself unto dust.

ANSARI OF HERAT

Love grows not in the field and is not sold in the market,
Whosoever would have it, whether king or beggar, must pay with his life.
Carry your head upon your palm as an offering,
If you would step into the Wonderland of love.

KABIR

Again:

Accursed be the life wherein one finds not love for the Lord;
Give your heart to His servant for He shall take you to Him.

Such self-surrender to the Master is only a prelude to the inheriting of a larger and purer Self than we otherwise know. Whosoever shall knock at its door is transformed into its own color:

A lover becomes the Beloved—such is the alchemy of his love;
God Himself is jealous of such a Beloved.

DADU

Calling on Ranjha, I myself become one with him.

BULLEH SHAH

LOVE AND THE LOVER'S RELATIONSHIP

It is of such a love that Lord Krishna spoke in the Gita, and of such a love that St. Paul preached to his listeners:

> *I am crucified with Christ; nevertheless I live; yet not I, but Christ liveth in me; and the life which I now live in the flesh I live by the faith of the Son of God, who loved me, and gave himself for me.*
>
> ST. PAUL

It is of this that the Sufis speak when they talk of *fana-fil-sheikh* (annihilation in the Master):

> *The vast expanse of myself is so filled to overflowing with the fragrance of the Lord that the very thought of myself has completely vanished.*

It is of this that the Christian mystics declare when they stress the necessity of "Death in Christ." As its initial phase, it may find analogies in earthly love, that between the parent and the child, friend and friend, lover and beloved, teacher and pupil, but once it has reached the point where the disciple discovers his teacher in his luminous glory within himself, all analogies are shattered and all comparisons are left behind; all that remains is a gesture, and then silence:

> *Let us write some other way*
> *Love's secrets—better so.*
> *Leave blood and noise and all of these*
> *And speak no more of Shamas Tabrez.*
>
> RUMI

XI. A PERFECT SCIENCE

EVEN THE FOREGOING BIRD'S-EYE SURVEY OF THE NATURE AND SCOPE OF THE SURAT SHABD YOGA CONVEYS SOME OF ITS UNIQUE FEATURES. He who studies it in relation to the other forms of yoga cannot but note the completeness of its solution of all the problems that confront the seeker when pursuing other systems. On the plane of outer action, it does not base itself on a dry and rigid discipline that is often laden with the consequences of psychological repression. It holds that some discipline is necessary, but adds that it must ultimately be inspired by inner spiritual experience and be a matter of spontaneous living, and not of rigorous asceticism and a too deliberate self-abnegation. The seeker must strive toward a state of equipoise and must therefore cultivate the virtue of moderation in thought and deed. The integration he thereby achieves enables him to gain greater concentration, and so higher inner experience, and this inner experience must in turn have repercussions on outer thoughts and action. The relationship of sadachar to inner sadhna is a reciprocal one; each enlivens and gives meaning to the other, and one without the other is like a bird with a single wing.

The Surat Shabd Yoga not only provides a means for achieving in practice the difficult ideal of sadachar, it also offers a mode of life that, while raising one above this physical world, does not enslave one to the realm of Name and Form. The Masters of this path know only too well that abstract speculations about the non-attributive aspect of the Absolute cannot lead one to It. How can man, conditioned by name and form, be drawn directly to that which is beyond name or form? Love seeks something which it can comprehend and to which it can attach itself, and God, if He is to meet man, must assume some shape or form. It is this recognition that inspires the devotion of the Bhakta to Shiva, Vishnu, Krishna, or Kali, the Divine Mother. But these divine beings represent fixed manifestations of God, and once the devotee has reached their plane, their very fixity, as we have seen already, prevents further progress. The Masters of the Surat Shabd Yoga wholly transcend this and all limitations by linking the seeker not to a fixed, but to an all-pervading manifestation of God: the Radiant Sound Current. It is this *anhat* and *anhad* Naam, this unstruck and unfathomable Word, that supports the various planes of creation ranging from pure spirit to gross matter. Its strains pervade every realm, every region, and it runs through them like a river that flows through the valleys which it has brought into being. And like the river, it exists in a fluid state, changing at every plane, yet ever remaining the same. The seeker who has been inspired by the love of the river of the Word is blessed indeed for he knows none of the limitations experienced by those who adore God in other forms. As he is drawn upward by Its beatific power, he finds It changing, modifying, becoming even stronger and purer, beckoning him on to higher and still higher effort, never allowing him to halt or to loiter, but leading him on from plane to plane, from valley to valley, until he arrives at the very source from where the Unmanifested comes into manifestation, the Formless assumes form, and the Nameless, name. It was this completeness of the inner journey made possible by the Yoga of the Sound Current that led Kabir to declare:

> *All holy ones are worthy of reverence,*
> *But I adore only one who has mastered the Word.*

APPENDIX

CHART OF THE CHAKRAS OR PLEXUSES

No.	Seat of the Ganglionic Centers	Presiding Deities (Hindu and Sufi)	Associated Elements	Representative Colors	Functions of Each Center	Merits of Meditation Thereon
1	Guda (rectum)	Ganesh	Earth	Yellow	Purification of the body	It rids one of all ailments and grants the capacity to fly in the air (levitation)
2	Indri (generative organ)	Brahma (Michael)	Water	Blue	Creation of species	Fearlessness, freedom from all bondage
3	Nabhi (navel)	Vishnu (Israel)	Fire	Red	Sustenance and preservation of species	Lord of all desires; heals all diseases; seer of hidden treasures; ability to enter into other bodies
4	Hirdey (heart)	Shiva (Gabriel)	Air	Bluish-white (smoky)	Disintegration, decay and death of species	The past, present and future reveal all their secrets
5	Kanth (throat)	Shakti (the Great Mother of the Universe)	Ether (all-pervading)	White (spotless)	The all-controlling power through the three Regents mentioned above with their specific functions	Enables one to become a yogishwar and knower of the Vedas, and to live a life of a thousand years
6	Aggya or Ajna (located behind and between the eyebrows with Antahkaran or the mind)	Atman — the disembodied spirit freed from all raiments	The active life principle; the very soul of Creation	Radiance and Luminosity in full splendor, ineffable	All in all, immanent in everything, the Alpha and Omega of all that is, visible and invisible	Confers the highest gift possible, with all powers, both natural and supernatural

SOME YAMAS AND NIYAMAS

	YAMAS	NIYAMAS
	Abstention from	*Acceptance and observance of*
1	Negation of God.	Faith in God and Godly power.
2	Self-indulgence.	Self-control and chastity (*Brahmcharya* or purity in thoughts, words and deeds).
3	Dishonest and fraudulent livelihood.	Earning a living by honest and truthful means.
4	Unhygienic and impure conditions of life, both within and without.	Cleanliness: inner, by water irrigation within and oxygenation, etc., and outer, by regular skin-baths, hip-baths, sun and air-baths, etc., and hygienic living conditions in sanitary surroundings.
5	Injuring others by thoughts, words and deeds (*himsa*).	Non-injury by thoughts, words and deeds (*ahimsa*).
6	Practicing falsehood, deceit and covetousness.	Cultivating truth, sincerity and charity.
7	Impatience, avarice and selfishness.	Patience, contentment and selfless service.
8	Self-assertion and ego-centricity.	Humility and self-surrender.

Daily Spiritual Diary

Observance	Failures	1	2	3	4	5	6	7	8	9	10	11	12	13	14	15	16	17	18	19	20	21	22	23	24	25	26	27	28	29	30	31	Total
Non-violence	In thought																																	
	In word																																	
	In deed																																	
Truthfulness	Falsehood																																	
	Deceit																																	
	Hypocrisy																																	
	Fraud																																	
	Illegal gain																																	
Chastity	In thought																																	
	In word																																	
	In deed																																	
Humility	Vanity of knowledge																																	
	Pride of wealth																																	
	Intoxication of power																																	
	Total																																	
Meditation	Meditation (Simran Dhyan)																																	
	Contacting the holy sound (Bhajan)																																	
	Total																																	
Selfless Service	Physically																																	
	Financially																																	

Extent of withdrawal from sensual consciousness.	Inner experience of vision.	Inner experience of hearing.	Any difficulty in meditation.	Daily Diary for month of _____ Name _____ Address _____

APPENDIX 63

TRADITIONAL HATHA YOGA FOODS

Foods conducive to the yogic sadhna	Foods that retard the yogic sadhna
1 Barley, black gram, whole mung (green gram), rice, til (gingelly seeds), shakar (jaggery), milk and milk products, butter and clarified butter — all in moderation.	Moth, mash, musur (lentils), peas, unhusked gram, wheat, oils and fats, sour milk and sour curd, spoiled ghee, meat in all forms, fish, fowl and eggs, etc.
2 Black pepper, almonds, ginger, currants, lime— in moderation.	Pineapple, red radishes.
3 Mangoes, grapes, guavas, apples, oranges, figs, gooseberries, dates and peaches, etc. — in moderation.	Watermelon and kakari.
4 Melon, cucumber — in small quantities.	Turi (snake gourd), kashiphal (red pumpkin), brinjal (eggplant), lady's finger and chulai (amaranth or spinach-like plant).
5 Pumpkin, plain turi (ridge gourd), ghia turi (plain gourd), spinach, parwal (coecinia indica) and swaran leaves — in small quantities.	Spices, condiments, chilies, pepper, sauces and other acid producing stimulants and things pungent, bitter and sour.

THE PLANES OF CREATION

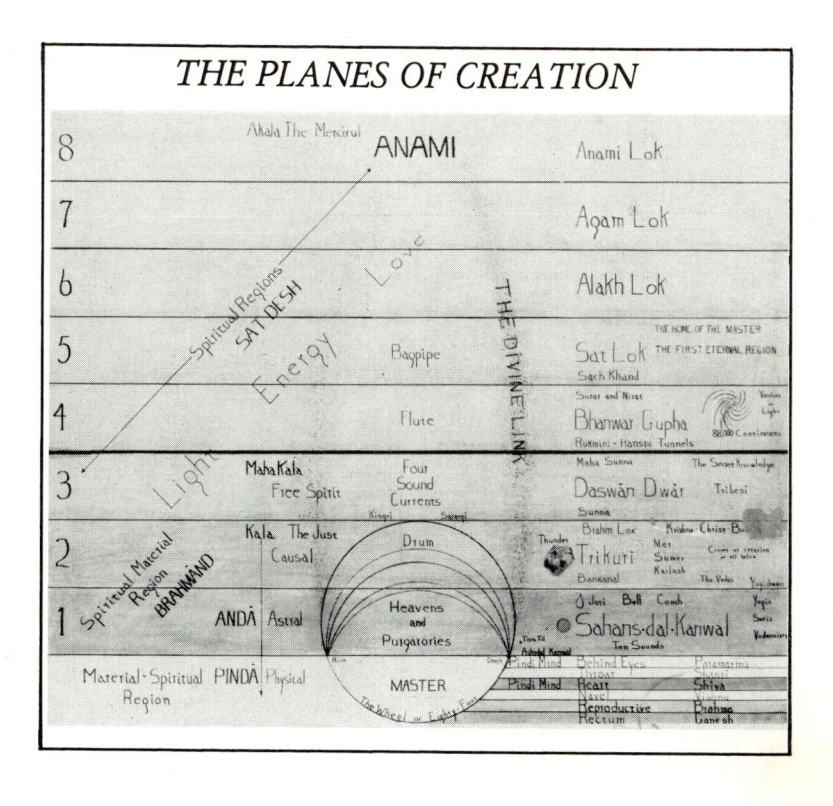

8		Akala The Merciful	ANAMI		Anami Lok
7					Agam Lok
6	Spiritual Regions	SAT DESH		THE DIVINE LINK	Alakh Lok
5		Love	Bagpipe		Sat Lok — THE HOME OF THE MASTER / THE FIRST ETERNAL REGION / Sach Khand
4	Energy		Flute		Sweet and Noisy / Bhanwar Gupha / Rukmini-Hansni Tunnels / Vortex / Light / 88,000 Continents
3	Light	MahaKala / Free Spirit	Four Sound Currents / Kingri / Sarangi		Maha Sunna / Daswan Dwar / Sunna / The Secret Knowledge / Triloni
2	Spiritual Material Region / BRAHMAND	Kala The Just / Causal	Drum	Thunder	Biahm Lok / Trikuti / Bansari / Krishna Christ Bu / Mer / Sumer / Kailash / Cause of creation of all below / The Vedas / Yogishan
1		ANDA / Astral	Heavens and Purgatories	Tara To / Ashabd Kanwal	Jyoti Bell Conch / Sahans-dal-Kanwal / Ten Sounds / Jogis / Saria / Videnisari
	Material · Spiritual / Region	PINDA / Physical	MASTER / The Wheel of Eighty Fou	Ruin / Pindi Mind	Pindi Mind / Behind Eyes / Throat / Heart / Navel / Reproductive / Rectum / Paramatma / Shiva / Vishnu / Brahma / Ganesh

APPENDIX 65

AFTERWORD

YOGA AND
THE OUTER SCIENCES

HAVING DISCUSSED IN SOME DETAIL THE VARIOUS METHODS OF YOGA, WE MAY IN CONCLUSION, REMIND OURSELVES OF THE TRUE WARNING SOUNDED BY SHANKARA (788-838):

> The three-fold path; the path of the world, the path of desires, and the path of scriptures, far from giving the knowledge of Reality, keeps one perpetually bound in the prison-house of the Universe. Deliverance comes only when one frees himself from this iron chain.
>
> Liberation cannot be achieved except by the perception of the identity of the individual spirit with the Universal spirit. It can be achieved neither by yoga, nor by Sankhya, nor by the practice of religious ceremonies, nor by mere learning.
>
> SHANKARACHARYA

To bring up to date Shankara's message that True Knowledge is a matter of direct perception and not mere ceremony, ritual or inference, we may add that it cannot come through the outer sciences either. The discoveries of the modern physical sciences have indeed been spectacular, and have confirmed many of the views about the nature of the cosmos and of existence voiced by the yogic systems. They have established, beyond doubt, that everything in the universe is relative, and that all forms are fundamentally brought into existence by the interplay of positive and negative energies. These discoveries have led some to presume that physical sciences can and will lead us to the same knowledge that yogins in the past sought through yoga; that science will replace yoga and make it irrelevant.

A blind man, though he may not be able to see the sun, may yet feel its heat and warmth. His awareness of some phenomenon which he cannot directly perceive, may lead him to devise and perform a series of experiments in order to know its nature. These experiments may yield him a lot of valuable data. He may be able to chart more accurately, perhaps, than the normal man, the course of the sun, its seasonal changes and the varying intensity of its radiation. But can all this knowledge that he has gathered be a substitute for a single moment's opportunity to view the sun directly for himself?

As with the blind man and the man of normal vision, so too with the scientist and the yogin. The physical sciences may yield us a lot of valuable, indirect knowledge of the Universe and its nature, but this knowledge can never take the place of direct perception, for just as the blind man's inferential knowledge cannot get at the sun's chief attribute which is light, so too the scientist in his laboratory cannot get at the cosmic energy's chief attribute, which is Consciousness. He may know a great deal about the universe, but his knowledge can never add up to universal consciousness. This consciousness can only be attained through the inner science, the science of yoga, which by opening our inner eye, brings us face to face with the Cosmic Reality. He whose inner eye has been opened, no longer needs to rely on spiritual hearsay, the assertions of his teacher, or mere philosophic or scientific inference. He sees God for himself and that exceeds all proof. He can say with Christ, "Behold the Lord!" or with Guru Nanak, "The Lord of Nanak is visible everywhere," or with Sri Ramakrishna, "I see Him just as I see you—only very much more intensely" (when replying to Naren—as Vivekananda was then known—on his very first visit, in answer to his question: "Master, have you seen God?").